Bedtime Stories for Adults

By: Mindfulness Mastery

Story 1: A Walk Through the Clearing

"I don't know how long I had been walking for, but I was sure that I must be almost there. My friend said it would take an hour or so to get to the clearing, but I had budgeted for two hours because I knew I wanted to take my time walking. I hadn't brought a watch with me, but judging by how far the sun had moved since I started, I was sure it had been nearly two hours at this point. I felt the crunching of the gravel under my feet as I continued to follow the marked trail, and took my time in admiring the sights around me. Luscious greenery adorned the path on either side and every now and again, I would see a squirrel or a bird flutter away from the path and into the trees to avoid being seen by me. Of course, I would always pause and watch, enjoying the experience of being alone in the forest with these beautiful creatures.

As I continued walking, I could see the path beginning to widen up ahead. In the distance, I could hear the gentle rushing of water and I knew that I had arrived where I was meant to. Despite how excited I was, I slowed my pace even more, wanting to take in all of the sights that were arising before me. After a long, hard year of going through many of life's trials and tribulations, this was my first true break alone and I did not want to waste it worrying or drowning in the overwhelm of my reality. I paused for a moment and breathed in deeply, smelling the green air from the fresh forestry around me. I sighed, feeling the sun shining against my back as it continued to rise through the sky. It must have been around 11:30 AM, as I had hit the trail around 9:30 AM. The heat of the sun was beginning to grow warmer and the forest was slowly drying out for the day as the dew from the night before began to evaporate. I took another step forward, and then another, allowing the lull of the waterfall's sweet sound to draw me forward. As I did, the view of the clearing began to open in front of me.

The clearing was just as my friend had described it: there was a large grassy patch with a crystal clear body of water off to the right side. The trees grew around the edges of the grass, yet not too close to the waterfall. There was plenty of space to enjoy the view, or get into the waterfall should I desire. Around the edges of the waterfall, the trees rose high, although none were taller than the peak of the waterfall itself. The waterfall fell down from a sheer cliff, which clearly had trees lining the falling body of water on either side at the top as well. The clearing felt cozy, almost like a small den that had been carved out of the vast forest.

I walked closer to the waterfall, and as I did, I could see the frothy bubbles foaming around the water from where the waterfall was rushing into it. As I reached the water, I noticed footprints were still formed in the sand at the edges of the water from people who had been there recently and I felt a sense of comfort in knowing that this space was enjoyed by many. I, too, slipped my own shoes off and followed the footprints, walking around the edge of the water and finding myself next to the cliff, looking in behind the waterfall itself. There, a moist rock wall that had been smoothed by the moving water stood tall and strong. I admired the way the water looked and wondered if anyone had ever crawled in there before to see the water from the back. I gazed at the trail that may lead there, but decided against it as I worried it may be too difficult for me to do on my own, and knew that I was alone so if I needed help I would be in trouble. After a few more moments, I turned around and saw the lush green grass behind me, and gazed out into the clearing from the opposite angle from where I had walked in from. I followed my footprints back toward my shoes, taking my time and feeling the moist ground beneath my feet. The sun continued to shine down over the clearing, and I could feel it growing warmer with every passing moment.

When I reached my shoes again, I turned back toward the water and began breathing in deeply, and exhaling all of my breath as much as I could. I sat down and dipped my toes into the edge of the water, feeling how cool it was against my skin, and meditating on the sensation of peace that was wrapped all around me. As I looked into the water, I could not help but notice how grateful I was for some clarity in my life, even if that clarity was merely the clear water at the edge of the waterfall. I looked up into the waterfall itself and saw how the water was white with fury from rushing off the edge of the cliff so fast, and paused for a moment to reflect on the lesson before me. That was, no matter how chaotic things may get, and no matter how fast, hard, or long we may fall for, there is always the potential that we may end up resting at the edge of calmness after our journey. I realized there was no reason for me to hold so tightly to my stresses and worries when I could just as easily relax into the moment and trust that in the end, I could find my calmness once more.

Story 2: Falling for Her

Daisy lived up the street in her father's farmhouse where she often worked early in the morning feeding the chickens, milking the cows, and rounding up the farm boys to put them to work for the day. After she was done, she would head to the bus stop and await the bus to take her to school. Rusty lived out of the way a bit, in a trailer park where his father had raised him since his Mom left them when they were younger. He was a rugged boy with a heart of gold, although he didn't show his heart to many for fear of what could happen if people saw him as sensitive instead of strong. Each morning, Daisy would get on the bus and Rusty would have a seat casually available for her, and she would always sit next to him. They didn't talk much at school as Rusty was a year ahead, but each morning they would talk endlessly on the bus about their wonders and curiosities, often landing on questions about what life outside of their small farm town would be like. Rusty was eager to leave it all behind and start fresh, and Daisy wondered what it would be like, although she had hesitations.

When Rusty graduated, he talked at great length about leaving, yet he never actually did. Instead, he took a job at Daisy's Dad's farm and worked there for a year while Daisy continued going to school to graduate. Each morning, Rusty would arrive at the farm and the two would feed the chickens, milk the cows, and prepare the daily task lists for the rest of the workers. Rusty would then work through the day as Daisy went to school, and he would greet her when she got home. When his work was done, Daisy would always come out to say goodbye and then Rusty would leave for the evening.

After a year of doing this, Daisy finally graduated and Rusty was eager to get out of town. The two had been talking in great length about what they would do, yet they had never fully settled on a plan. Rusty wanted to move to Chicago, but Daisy was not ready to leave Oklahoma. Over time, Rusty worried that he may have to move away and leave Daisy behind. It was around this time that Rusty realized that he had fallen deeply in love with Daisy, as he could not imagine leaving her behind and living a life without her. Daisy had not said anything, but she, too, was terrified of Rusty leaving and forgetting about her as she had also fallen in love with Rusty. Still, the two could not decide what it was that they wanted to do.

When the day came that Daisy graduated, Rusty came to her graduation and stood off in the distance so Daisy's father wouldn't see him there. Daisy got excited upon seeing Rusty there, and immediately after the ceremony rushed over to see him. To her surprise, Rusty wrapped his arms around her, kissed her forehead, and congratulated her for graduating. He spun her around in a circle, cheering for her and enjoying this moment of finally getting to hold her close. They both felt the depth of their love growing as they embodied this moment together. When they were done, Daisy went back to see her family and celebrated with them at a local diner before heading back to the farm.

The next day, Rusty arrived at the farm, only this time his car was packed full of his belongings. Daisy's heart sank as she realized what was happening, so she stayed in the house, as she did not want to have to say goodbye. She watched out the window as Rusty talked to her father and let him know it was time for him to go, and Daisy's father shook Rusty's hand. Rusty then looked toward the house and caught a glimpse of Daisy in the window. He waved to her to come out, but Daisy was sad and instead sat down at the kitchen table and stirred a spoonful of sugar into her tea. Rusty came into the house, much to her surprise, and asked Daisy to go with him to Chicago and live their lives together, like he knew they were meant to do. Daisy frowned and said she could not leave her family, especially without knowing when she would be able to see them again. Rusty had it all figured out, though, as he dropped an envelope on the table in front of her. "That's enough money for you to buy a bus ticket home if you decide you don't want to be with me in Chicago anymore, and I'll bring you back here every other month for a visit, I promise. Will you come?" Rusty asked. Daisy smiled, picked up the envelope, and decided she would give it a try.

Years went by and Daisy and Rusty continued living in Chicago and visiting their families in Oklahoma every other month. Daisy never used the bus fare to return home, but eventually, she did use it to buy a new cradle for their first born baby. Together, Daisy and Rusty raised a family of three children, two cats, and a dog in their home in Chicago. They spent each day talking about the wonders of the world, reminiscing on their days at the farm, and enjoying each other's company.

One day, Daisy's father died and he had left his farm behind for Daisy to keep. Together, Daisy and Rusty decided to relocate their family back to the old farm where they picked up where they had left off years before, as if they had never skipped a beat. Their kids took the bus to school, and on that bus, their eldest daughter Rosie fell in love with a boy named Evan from the trailer park up the road. Daisy and Rusty often smiled as they looked out at their kids boarding the bus, recalling the days when they themselves were just teenagers falling in love.

Story 3: College Sweethearts

When Carole and Jordon were freshmen in college, they met at a coffee cart outside of the main entrance to the old campus lot. Their meeting was like one straight out of a storybook, complete with cool fall weather, colorful leaves strewn about, and cozy scarves, and toques adorning everyone to help them stay warm. One morning in the fall of freshman year, Carole was standing with her friends in line at the coffee cart and Jordon was working the cart to earn some extra cash to help purchase new filming equipment. When Carole was next in line, she walked up to the cart and ordered an Americano with extra whip cream. "Odd order," Jordon answered, scribbling it down on a piece of paper. "Whip cream on coffee?" He asked. "Just the way I like it." Carole smiled, handing Jordon exact change for her drink. As she handed him the change, Carole and Jordon locked eyes and smiled, pausing for a moment to take in the simple and sweet beauty of falling in love with each other.

Carole thought Jordon was attractive, so she made a mental note of which cart he was working at and came back to that cart each morning for weeks after. Some mornings, Jordon would be working and he would prepare her drink for her. Others, he would not be working but he would always seem to be nearby the cart so that when she was done ordering they could share some conversation before they each parted ways to attend their respective classes. Without ever telling the other, the two of them always did their best to ensure that they would see each other every single morning.

Carole and Jordon grew fond of their morning conversations. They also started getting braver and braver as they each began leaving little hints about having an attraction toward the other. Carole would always smile and give Jordon a hug if he was not working, and Jordon would always draw little smiley faces or hearts on Carole's Americano with the whipped cream. These two lovers had a great deal of fun falling for each other and enjoy casually flirting with one another each morning before classes.

One day, during the middle of winter, when it was particularly cold outside, Jordon proposed that the two of them head inside and grab a bite to eat. It just so happened that Carole did not have to be at class for another forty-five minutes, so she agreed and the two of them walked together to the cafeteria hall to eat their breakfasts with each other. They spent the entire time laughing, enjoying each other's company, and falling even more deeply in love with each other.

When the breakfast was done, the two parted ways and went to their respective classes. All morning, they both found themselves distracted by thoughts of the other. They loved how it felt so normal to be with each other, and how spending time together seemed to come so easily. When their classes were over that day, Carole went back to her dorm to study. At some point that evening, she heard a knock at her door. When she answered it, she saw none other than Jordon standing there, smiling, with his hands stuffed in his pockets. He paused for a moment before asking if she wanted to go to the library with him to study together, and Carole happily agreed. The two of them spent the evening studying, joking, and enjoying each other's company.

After that, Carole and Jordon began hanging out almost daily. They would share breakfast, study sessions, or even just walks around the campus as they enjoyed each other's presence. When spring break came, they carpooled back to see their family as they both came from the same small town in Connecticut. They would listen to their favorite songs on the ride back home, sing, laugh, and spend even more time getting to know each other along the way.

As the years went by, Carole and Jordon became inseparable. In sophomore year, they spent spring break on a vacation together in Cape Cod where they enjoyed delicious seafood dinners and beach walks together each evening. In junior year, they spent Christmas at each other's family's houses, enjoying two dinners, and sharing the opportunity to meet each other's extended families. By senior year, they fell so deeply in love that there was no way these two could be separated from each other's company.

When graduation was right around the corner, Jordon began acting strange. Carole thought he was reconsidering their relationship since college would be over soon and became worried that the love of her life was preparing to leave her. Jordon became scared because he had no idea what the love of his life would think about him wanting to spend the rest of their lives together. Shortly after the two walked across the stage, Jordon got down on one knee and proposed to Carole. He proposed that she marry him, that they move in together, that they start their careers, and that they eventually have the children and dogs that they always dreamed about having during their late night study sessions. Carole cried as she realized that Jordon had been acting weird because he was about to propose, not because he was preparing to leave her. She said yes, and the two cried together as they celebrated the reality that they would go on to live the rest of their lives together. The two lived happily ever after, as they say in the fairy tales.

Story 4: The Peaceful Path

Gary was a forty-something-year-old man who had been working for the same office job for nearly twenty years now. He was a busy man with many meetings every day, bosses who had high expectations of him and a family at home who regularly demanded more of his time and attention than he felt he had to give. Gary always strived to be everything his family, boss, and friends wanted and needed him to be, yet he never felt like he could keep up. Often, he would find himself standing in the shower at the beginning of what would be a very long day attempting to wash away his troubling thoughts. Gary felt like his mind was racing all the time, and sometimes in the shower was his only opportunity to clear his thoughts so that he could feel at peace with himself. It never lasted, but for those few moments in the shower in between thoughts of what he had to get done that day he would feel fleeting sensations of relief.

One day, Gary went into work and it became too much for him to handle. He was already feeling guilty about missing his Mom's birthday dinner because of needing to be at work, so when his boss started yelling at him, Gary couldn't take it anymore. He found himself in the bathroom with the door locked, talking himself out of a panic attack, and trying to find a moment of peace. He realized this was happening more and more: he would become overwhelmed with the demands of life and be desperate to feel even a fleeting moment of peace in between the stress. Despite how hard he wished for it, Gary could never seem to find the peace that he was looking for.

Gary searched everywhere for the peace he desired. He tried buying the things that he believed would bring him peace, but all they did was cause him to feel sad when it didn't work. He tried to create peace by purchasing expensive vacation packages for his family, but all he felt was stressed over the added expenses that he had to incur. He tried to talk to local yogis and meditation guides to try and find out how to get peace into his life, and while he understood the logic behind all of their teachings, Gary would not allow himself to actually do what the guides said. Instead, he would write off their suggestions as being "too easy" and then he would begin going about his life as usual.

Gary spent years upon years trying to find out how he could find peace, and eventually, he gave up. He became so fed up that the methods he was trying were not working that he decided peace must be an illusion and that everyone claiming to have it must be lying. Gary became so angry with all of the yogis and meditation guides in his town that any time he heard someone talk about them he would frown, claim that peace was a load of nonsense and that it was unattainable, and then end the conversation or leave.

One day, Gary became so angry with his failure to find peace and his deep-seated need for experiencing peace, that he threw his hands up in the air and admitted defeat. He was in his car after work, sitting in the grocery parking lot, and he was truly angry after being cussed out by his boss for the duration of the day. To put it simply, Gary was fed up with his life and he had reached the point where he could no longer take it. With his hands in the air, Gary yelled at the skies out of the front window of his car. "I can't take it anymore!" He shouted, dropping his fists into his lap and leaning his head over the steering wheel. "I can't take the stress, the demands, the overwhelm. I love my family and I can't even handle them anymore! It's too much!" He muttered, feeling his eyes flooding hot with tears. Now, this was a big deal for Gary. Gary was a very proud man, he was so proud that he rarely showed his anxiety, stress, or anger to anyone else. So, for Gary to be sobbing out all of his pent up stress in his car was a big deal.

After several minutes of sobbing in his car and releasing the stress that he had been carrying around inside of him, Gary found that there were no tears left. Almost suddenly, he no longer had the fear of what he had been holding on inside of him anymore, there was no sadness or stress left to be experienced in that moment. Gary sat up, wiped his eyes, and looked around his car to make sure that no one had seen him lose it in the grocery store parking lot. When he realized he was alone, and that all of his emotions had been felt, Gary felt a surge of peace rush through him. Just like that, he found what he had been looking for all along. In that moment, Gary realized that peace was not something that he could buy, manufacture, or obtain. Instead, peace was an emotion like any other, and it could be experienced and expressed through allowing himself to just be.

From that day forward, Gary made a routine of allowing himself private space to feel and express his emotions to himself. This way, he could continue to hold his pride around his family, without carrying the burden of his stress with him, too. As a result, Gary became a happier, healthier, and more peaceful man overall. He even joined a few of those meditation classes and followed some local yogi's through their practices as he learned to cultivate even more peace from within.

Story 5: Priorities

Jack was a 65-year-old man who was rather proud of the life that he had built for his family. He had worked hard since his teenage years and done everything he could over the past five decades to give his family the life that he felt they deserved. He spent long hours working as a laborer, pulling in as many extra shifts as he could so that he could provide for his family. Thanks to his hard work, his wife was able to stay home and raise their three children in a beautiful home that he had purchased for them. He filled the home full of furniture, food, and various treasures based on whatever his family desired to have. When his family wanted to go on vacation, he would work overtime to afford the added expense and would always plan dreamy vacations that brought his family great joy. They would visit places like Disney Land, Martha's Vineyard, and even Arizona to see the desert. His family traveled to many different places enjoying all of the different views and creating many different memories.

Although he seemed to be around fairly frequently, Jack never felt as though he was able to truly relax and enjoy his time with his family. He had grown so used to working hard that he always had to be doing something: fixing something, building something, cleaning something, or moving something around.

No matter what day it was or how much work he had already done, Jack would always do more work than what was reasonable because he simply felt uncomfortable just sitting around and enjoying the presence of his family. To Jack, nothing felt more satisfying than retiring after a hard day of working and feeling the comfort of his pillow rising to meet him.

One day, when he turned 66, Jack found that he was not feeling as good as he used to. For a while, he chalked it up to being older and dealing with regular pains of old age. After a few months, however, Jack could no longer deny that he was experiencing some fairly serious symptoms. His symptoms had grown so strong that he could no longer do the labor work that he once had, so he quit his job and retired to please his family. If it were up to him, Jack would have found a way to keep working despite his setbacks with his health. Still, he listened and retired, as he knew he probably should.

Shortly into his retirement, even simple things became challenging for Jack. He could no longer work like he used to, and eventually, even smaller tasks like climbing the stairs or going for a walk to the mailbox became more of a challenge for him. Finally, with his family's insistence, Jack went to visit a doctor to see why he might be experiencing such hardship with his health. It was from that appointment that Jack went on to learn that he was terminally ill with cancer and that he had waited too long to be checked so he was beyond the point of being able to be cured.

Jack and his family were shocked by this news as they realized that the once vital and virile man was quickly falling apart before their very eyes. Within weeks, Jack could no longer climb the stairs at all, and sometimes he even had troubles holding his coffee mug or pouring himself a glass of water. His wife, Susan, had to do everything for him. Being unable to do anything for himself made Jack angry and embarrassed, as he had always been a very proud and self-sufficient man. He spent the past five decades taking care of this woman; he did not feel as though he needed his wife to be taking care of him, now.

As time went on, Jack's anger turned into sadness. His family would all visit him in his home and bring their young children around, and everyone would play and get along like they always had. This time, though, Jack was forced to sit there and observe and partake in the conversation as he could no longer get up and find some work to do to keep himself busy. It was during these visits that Jack grew to understand just how much he had missed by being so deeply devoted to his work ethic and not spending enough time paying attention to his family. He realized that he had missed countless birthdays, holidays, anniversaries, and even just simple day-to-day memories because he was so absorbed in his need to work that he never truly sat down to enjoy his family until it was almost too late.

At first, Jack was angry with himself for not having spent more time with his family. He could not understand how foolish he had been by working so intensely and missing out on the majority of his children's and grandchildren's lives. Then, he became angry that he felt he had no choice but to work that hard to be able to give them the life that he wanted them all to enjoy. Eventually, Jack found himself thanking his own life for giving him enough time to see what he had missed and for giving him the opportunity to make up for it now before it was too late.

One day, when he was talking to his son, Jack decided to offer him some advice about his work ethic. Jack said, "Son, when I was your age my priorities were all wrong. I thought I had to work the hardest, be the best, and make the most money to make my family happy. Your mother told me she wanted me around more and wished I was there for the kids more, and I justified my actions by saying that I was there financially to support them. But that's not enough, son. In life, simply giving someone our money and hard work is not enough. If you truly want to be happy and live your best life, you take some time every single day to sit with those kids of yours and enjoy them. Never work so hard that you miss birthdays, anniversaries, or even just those special suppers each night. Be there for as many moments as you can, son, because believe me, one day they will have all slipped by. I realize now my priorities were wrong, and I taught you wrong. The true priority you need to have in life is to be able to provide for your family, but not just with finances. Prioritize the opportunity to provide them with your time, your attention, and your love. Believe me, son. It will make a world of difference."

Jack's son never forgot this story and went on to live by these words even long after Jack had passed. In fact, Jack's son went on to teach his own children about the value of these priorities, and they went on to teach their children! So, thanks to Jack and his hard work, his entire family was able to enjoy more quality time together for generations to come because he took the time to realize that prioritizing finances was not the only important thing in life. Time, attention, and love also mattered when it comes to providing for your family and truly taking care of them, and yourself.

Story 6: Values

Sarah was an average small town girl, raised in a farming community in the southern states. For as long as Sarah could remember, she always dreamed about leaving the small community and heading out to the big city to enjoy a fast-paced lifestyle. Sarah would dream about hopping in her car when she was 18, heading off to college, and then starting a career in a big city like New York or Los Angeles. She would draw pictures of it and hang it on her wall, dream about it, and talk about it any chance she got. Her parents were sad that Sarah wanted to leave so badly, so they always did their best to show Sarah the value of living in a small community. They did this by teaching Sarah how to establish friendships with her neighbors, how to become self-sufficient, and how to market herself so that she could share their family business with their neighbors. Sarah's parents ran a produce store from their farm, so Sarah gained great business knowledge from her years spent working on the farm.

Despite how hard her parents tried to keep her from leaving when she turned 18, Sarah simply could not wait to leave for college and then start her city life. Just as she always planned, she packed up her belongings in her car and left for college. Sarah spent four years getting her business degree so that she could move to New York and work for corporate America. Although her parents did not fully understand her dreams, they always showed their support in helping Sarah get to where she wanted to go.

As Sarah emerged into the corporate world, she realized that her business education did not offer her enough on its own to help her succeed. In fact, her business degree gave her the knowledge needed to get the jobs, but it was really her small town values that gave Sarah what she needed to get hired. Because she had been raised to value friendship and community, and to share her services and market her business boldly with the world around her, Sarah learned how to have good business sense.

It was through truly working in New York and acquiring these jobs using the charisma and values that her parents instilled in her that allowed her to truly understand the value of her upbringing. As she was sitting in her corner office admiring the view and eating lunch one day, Sarah realized just how much her parents had contributed to her being able to get to where she was. She realized that if it were not for her small town values, Sarah would have never made the impact she was meant to have in the city. In fact, she may have failed and ended up right back at her parents' house, pursuing something she did not love and living a life that she did not want.

Although her parents did not fully understand, Sarah silently thanked them every single day for raising her in a small town and giving her those values. She no longer resented them for keeping her in that small town and preventing her from living a big city life as a kid. Instead, she was grateful for the entire experience. Sarah still had no desire to move back to the small town that she grew up in, but she did hold it in higher esteem as she realized that it was this small town and her family that had gotten her to where she was, not just her and her schooling.

In life, having values and sharing values is important. When we learn how to care about the things that matter, these core values stay with us for life and they help us in ways we cannot possibly imagine until we are in those situations. There is nothing more valuable than knowing what your own values are and using those values to support you in creating your dream life. So, do not be afraid to dream big and forge a new path for yourself, but also do not forget to honor where you came from and the values that you were taught by the people who raised you.

Story 7: Passion

Darlene was a forty-something-year-old woman who had spent her entire life doing everything that she knew she was supposed to do. She woke up every morning at six to feed her dogs and her cat, she made breakfast for her children and her husband, and she fixed a pot of morning coffee. When everyone was fed, she would clean their plates away, tidy up the kitchen, and help everyone get ready for their day. Then, it was off to school. Darlene would then head into the office to work until the school day was over. She would then go pick up her children, bring them home, feed them a snack, and escort them to their after-school activities like soccer, dance, and swim lessons. When everyone got home in the evening, Darlene would fix up a supper, feed everyone, and then clean all of the dishes when everyone was done eating. She would then clean up everyone's book bags and shoes, tidy up any other messes that had been made that day, and then sit down to watch thirty minutes of television before bed. On weekends, Darlene would do all of the same things except instead of going to school or work she would take her kids shopping, to sleepovers, or to their sports events. There was always something going on, and Darlene was always in charge of having to make sure that everything got done in time.

When she was in her early forties, Darlene realized that she was entirely miserable. After spending nearly two decades cleaning up after her family, preparing meals for them, and driving them around everywhere, Darlene realized that she was done. She no longer cared to have the experience of doing everything herself, as it was beginning to take a toll on her. She found that every morning she would wake up depressed and dreading the day before her, and every night she would go to sleep sad and wishing that she could wake up to a brand new life. This brought Darlene great guilt as she loved her family and loved caring for them, though she could no longer do it all by herself.

One day, Darlene was called into her boss's office in the middle of the afternoon. As she got up from her desk and headed toward her bosses office, Darlene tried to recall anything she may have done wrong that could result in her being talked to or written up by her boss. Of course, she could not think of anything she had done wrong as Darlene was always very particular about doing everything properly and by the book. After all, she was great at doing what she knew was expected of her. When she reached her bosses office, Darlene's boss asked her to sit and offered to get her a beverage. Darlene agreed and began sipping on the tea that her boss had brought her as she tried to understand what it was that she had been called in for. To her surprised, Darlene's boss offered her a promotion that came with a substantial raise and increased benefits compared to what she was already receiving. Darlene was excited by the offer, but at the same time, she was miserable to realize that taking it meant that she would be committing to staying in this lackluster life that she was no longer getting joy from. Before she knew what she was doing, Darlene refused the promotion and instead put in her notice and quit her job. She went and cleared out her desk and left, never to look back again.

Darlene's family was surprised to learn that she had quit her job and had no intentions of going back. They were also surprised when she said that she would no longer make breakfast unless she felt like it, that everyone would need to find their own ways to their hangouts, and that the only thing Darlene would help with anymore was getting to sports events or homework. At this point, her kids were old enough that they could walk, bike, or even drive themselves to their own events so she would no longer have to do it. In other words, Darlene was ready to start letting her children grow up and become young adults.

Asserting these boundaries meant that Darlene had great freedom in her life to do whatever it was that she pleased. She could sleep in, eat whenever she wanted, and even watch afternoon television shows that she had heard her friends talking about at the PTA meetings at her children's school for years. Finally, Darlene got what it meant to slow down and just be, rather than to always have to be in motion doing everything in her power to please everyone else.

At first, Darlene's laid back lifestyle was enjoyable as it offered her a great change of pace from what she was used to. Over time, however, it grew boring as she realized that she would always be doing nothing unless she did something to change that. As she did not want to spend her entire life bored, Darlene began looking into different hobbies and discovering new things that she liked. One hobby she found that she was drawn to was making jewelry. Darlene found that not only did she enjoy making jewelry, but also that she was incredibly good at it, and that people often wanted to purchase her jewelry.

Darlene started out making jewelry as a hobby in the afternoons while she watched daytime television. She would make four or five new pieces per week, and inevitably every single piece would sell to someone that she knew. Eventually, she started selling her jewelry online as this gave her the opportunity to sell even more. Before she knew it, Darlene was making copious amounts of jewelry and selling them to friends, family, strangers online, and even stocking it in boutique stores around her town. She grew so excited to make jewelry that Darlene would excitedly get up in the middle of the night and sketch out new plans, or launch from bed in the morning ready to start crafting new creations.

Although it was a far cry from what she was used to, Darlene loved her new life of making and selling handmade jewelry. Her children and husband liked it as well, as they began to realize that Darlene was happier and enjoying life once again. It took them some time to get used to Darlene not being available to help as often anymore, but in the end, they were all happy that Darlene had found her passion and that she was finally enjoying life after helping her family do the very same thing for so many years.

Story 8: Tranquility

It was four in the afternoon on a Saturday, and the sun was perched lazily above the trees. I had grown bored of sitting in my house, so I decided to walk to the local park and sit at a bench instead and watch people around me enjoying their lives. When I arrived, the park was bustling with young families playing, lovers holding hands, and individuals jogging or biking around the parameter of the park. It was a busy day, as everyone was enjoying the late summer sunshine before it went away for another season.

All around, people were enjoying the day as much as they could. When I had sat down, I admired a few young families that were running around together playing Frisbee. Their younger children were running wild, without a care in the world. It was clear that they were too young to truly understand the concept of Frisbee; so instead, they chased their parents around the grass and laughed each time they would turn on their heels and tumble to the ground. The older children were rather competitive, fighting over who was scoring the most points and who would come out as the winner of this game of Frisbee. The parents were playing, although they were playing with much less concern than the children. They did not care who was winning or losing, they were simply helping show their children how to throw the Frisbee and catch it properly.

In another direction, a lovely couple had arrived and were holding hands and giggling as they slowly followed the path through the park. They were not making much grounds, as they would stop every so often to hug, kiss, and enjoy each other's presence. The smiles on their faces said it all, as they were clearly in the process of falling deeply in love with each other. I smiled as they continued walking through the park without a care in the world for anyone or anything around them. I remembered back to when my wife and I were younger and falling in love, and I quietly thanked them for bringing back these long since gone memories to my elderly mind. I smiled at the thought of how beautiful it was to enjoy such times together with our loved ones.

As I leaned back on the bench, a young man jogged in front of me, making his way down the trail. He seemed to be listening to some fairly loud music as he ran by, likely to help keep him focused and make the process more enjoyable. I watched as he breathed rhythmically, keeping his breaths focused and making steady progress through the park. Eventually, he reached the end of the trail and took off down the sidewalk, likely heading back home from his afternoon jog.

As I sat in the park and looked around me, I realized that all around me life was bustling and yet I was sitting, undisturbed, in my quiet little space on the bench. Every now and again someone would smile and wave at me as they walked past, but otherwise, I was simply alone and enjoying the moment. I closed my eyes for a brief moment and breathed in deeply, smelling the sweet summer air that was all around. When I opened them up again, I took a moment to look past all of the people and see the park itself. Trees edged the pathway on the distant side of the park, and only grass and small bushes here and there lined it the rest of the way. There were benches every so often, as well as a few garbage cans with waste stations for people who had brought their dogs around. Behind me, a luscious community garden was rich with flowers and vegetables. It was filled with bumble bees and butterflies that were enjoying the gentle breeze that helped them glide from flower to flower, and plant to plant.

I sat for several more minutes, enjoying the tranquility of the moment and feeling into the peace of it all. In my younger years, times like this did not mean much to me. I was more likely to be the couple laughing and falling in love, or the Dad teaching his children how to throw a Frisbee through the park so that they could enjoy a fun game together. I may have even been the man jogging at one point, far before I had ever met my wife or had kids with her. It was fascinating to see the tranquil reality of all different stages of life spread out before me.

When I was done sitting, I grabbed my cane from the bench and stood up, placing it on the ground beneath my feet. I could hear the gravel crunching beneath my feet and cane as I slowly made my way back home, where I would sit in the living room and admire the pictures of my wife and kids and remember the life we once shared together. There, I would be alone too, and I would experience an entirely different type of tranquil compared to the lively and bright one at the park.

Story 9: Forgiveness

Chloe and Joy had been friends for many years. They grew up in the same town together, with their houses right next door to each other. They met when they were around four years old, when Joy moved in next to Chloe. For years, the two of them would play together, running around the neighborhood playing tag, pretending that sticks were their swords, and playing in Chloe's backyard treehouse. The two were practically inseparable, as they rode the bus to school together, went to the same class, played together after school, and slept over at each other's houses all the time. When they reached high school, they had some classes together and some classes apart, yet they still spent the majority of their time together. They would spend lunch hour together talking about their homework and boys, get ready for school together in the morning, and carpool to school each day. On weekends, they attended their boyfriend's sporting events or the party of the weekend, or they would simply catch a movie together. To put it simply, they did everything together.

When they graduated, Chloe and Joy were excited to attend college together. They had both applied at all of the same colleges and universities and had agreed that they would go to a school together and share an apartment off campus together, as they had dreamed of this their entire lives. In senior year while they were applying to colleges and universities, they also found that a few other things in their lives were changing. Joy had met a boy who she really liked and started dating, and the two started hanging out more frequently. Chloe grew frustrated when Joy was no longer hanging out with her, but Joy knew that Chloe would get over it eventually. Unfortunately, Chloe never did get over it. The argument grew even more complicated when Joy chose to go to the same school as her boyfriend rather than the same school as Chloe, and Chloe could not attend that school, as she had not been accepted.

When they graduated and left for college, Joy, and Chloe were not even talking anymore as Chloe was so hurt by Joy's actions. Joy was sad that Chloe was hurt, but was also frustrated that Chloe was not being supportive of Joy's romance and desires to make her own path in life. The two were so frustrated at each other that they hardly talked through freshman and sophomore year. However, in junior year they were both at home at the same time and crossed each other's paths in the driveway. Chloe was mad, but Joy wanted to reconcile. She did her best to explain to Chloe what had happened and that she was sorry, but Chloe was not interested in hearing what Joy had to say. She ignored Joy and walked to her car and took off, and Joy hardly ever saw Chloe after that. From that day forward, the two never connected when they were at home, even if they saw each other outside they would just pretend that the other did not exist.

One day after they had both graduated, Joy's family decided to sell the family home and move away to a new state. Joy no longer returned back to the family home, which meant that she never had the potential of running into Chloe in the driveway anymore. In a way, she was relieved that she would not have to run into that awkward encounter anymore. In another way, Joy was upset that it felt like she would never have the chance to reconcile with her old best friend. She knew that after her family sold and moved away, it was unlikely that she would ever be able to get back in touch with her friend, which meant that the relationship was officially over, for good.

Chloe was also sad when she saw that Joy's family had moved. For her, knowing that Joy would always be there or coming back was comforting, as she knew that there would always be the chance that the two of them would reconcile and save their friendship. After Joy's family had moved, it became apparent that this chapter was officially closed. Chloe was disappointed in herself for not treating Joy better and for being unwilling to see the whole reality, as this lead to Joy thinking that Chloe was unwilling to reconcile the relationship.

For years, as the two grew their careers, raised their families, and lived their separate lives, they both experienced intense guilt around the end of their relationship. Both women wished that they had contributed to finding reconciliation more so that they could have lived their lives together. They missed calling each other and sharing moments together and always wished that they could have grown together through these later parts of life. Despite the fact that Joy went on to marry her high school sweetheart whom she went to college with, she always wished that she would have chosen to go to school with Chloe or put more effort into keeping their friendship alive. Chloe always wished that she had not been so stubborn and that she had been willing to see things from Joy's perspective, especially once she realized that Joy and her now husband's relationship was serious. At the time, Chloe thought it would be a short term fling and felt betrayed by Joy's lack of loyalty, but she no longer saw it this way. Still, it felt like it was too late for them to reconcile, so they both kept their guilt to themselves and refused to do anything about it.

One day, Joy was walking through the grocery store when she saw a familiar face. "Chloe? Is that you?" She asked, walking up to the lady by the fruit. "Joy?" Chloe asked, shocked. "I thought you family left this area?" She asked, looking at Joy. "They did, but Ronald and I moved back recently." Joy smiled. The two talked in the produce section of the grocery store for nearly an hour before swapping numbers and agreeing to meet up with each other. They both apologized for their actions and forgave each other, realizing now that their feud had gone on far too long and that the consequences were far harsher than the action itself. The ladies realized that their friendship was strong and that there was no amount of time or space that could prevent them from being each other's best friends.

Over the next several weeks, they caught each other up on their lives and began hanging out again on a regular basis. They talked as if nothing had changed, and they spent plenty of time together bonding once again. They realized that they had believed forgiveness would be harder than it truly was and that they had both lost a lot of time with each other due to their unwillingness to forgive each other. From that day forward, Chloe and Joy remained best friends. They also learned that if they were ever going through something with a loved one, it was better to find a way to reconcile and to mend the relationship, rather than allowing years of guilt and hurt to pass first.

Story 10: Joy

Ruth was an elderly lady now, in her mid-seventies. She sat on her patio each morning, overlooking the neighborhood and waving to the people as they walked by. Each morning, children would walk to school and families would walk their dogs, and Ruth would just watch and smile at each one. This time of day was Ruth's favorite, as it reminded her of all of the wonderful things that she had to be joyful about in her lifetime.

Ruth remembered her childhood when she would walk to school with her six siblings and enjoy classes at the schoolhouse. She was not very fond of her teachers, but she loved learning and she loved playing outside with her friends on breaks. She remembered sitting in the grass one afternoon eating a snack her Mom had packed for her and watching the younger kids play hopscotch in the dirt. To Ruth, this was one of her favorite memories that she shared with her siblings because it was so simple and brought so much joy to her life.

Ruth also remembered when she graduated and met her husband, Donald. Donald went straight into the military after school and served the country for nearly half a decade. For that entire time, Ruth raised their family, took care of the home front, and sent letters to Donald every week as she let him know how much she loved him and missed him. She would pour the day to day happenings into the letters, always trying to give Donald a feel of what was going on at home so that he felt like he was not missing out when he was gone. She remembered the sheer joy of seeing Donald for the first time, and for the first time after he returned home from every deployment. It always felt like she was falling in love all over again when he returned home.

Ruth also remembered what it felt like when Donald finally came home and stayed home, as he was done serving in the military. She remembered waking up to him every single day, learning how to live together as a couple, and living in sheer awe of this man who she adored so much. Ruth found so much joy in seeing Donald every day that she always did her best to find the small ways to bring even more joy into their days on a regular basis. Whether it was brewing him coffee when he was tired or slow dancing with him in the kitchen, Ruth loved bringing a smile to Donald's face in any way that she could.

As an older couple walked by holding hands, Ruth remembered the joy she gained from holding hands with Donald all through his life. When they were walking in public, he would always grab her hand in his and lead her around, which helped Ruth feel so cared for and protected. She remembered how strong his hand felt, and how his body always seemed to be positioned in a way where he was ready to protect her if she needed him. Donald was a very protective and caring man, and Ruth always felt so safe in his presence.

Ruth remembered how even when Donald was ill with cancer, he was still so strong and protective until he could no longer be. As he withered away and he found that he was no longer able to physically protect Ruth, he still did his best to mentally and emotionally protect her by comforting her and telling her that everything would be okay. Donald told Ruth how he would watch over her every day so that she could carry on without him, even when she believed that she would never be able to. She was to wake up every day and continue looking for joy in every day, just as she had done since he had come home from the war. Donald told Ruth that she was to brew herself coffee, dance to their favorite songs while she sang quietly to herself, and walk with bravery everywhere she went. This, Donald said, would be the way that she could feel his presence after he left.

Now, nearly twenty years after he had passed, Ruth still found ways to bring herself joy every morning. Part of that joy was in brewing herself a fresh pot of Donald's favorite coffee every morning and sipping a cup on the porch while she watched the families go by, while reminiscing on her own family that had long since grown and left. At night, she would put on their favorite songs and dance, or sing to them as she wiped off her makeup and prepared herself for bed.

As she was preparing to head inside for the day, Ruth saw an elderly couple walking their grandchildren to school. This made Ruth reminisce on her own grandchildren, and what it was like when they visited. When her children came to visit her, Ruth would share her favorite memories of Donald with them, in hopes of keeping his memory alive and introducing him to his grandkids through her memories. She would show them his photographs and watch them in sheer awe of how joyful they were to get to know the man that she had once loved so dearly, and in that she would find joy of her own. Every time, she knew that Donald was right there smiling with them and holding her hand, helping her stay brave whenever she missed him the most.